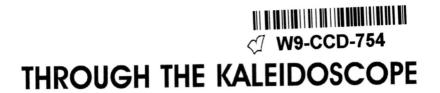
THROUGH THE KALEIDOSCOPE

VIEWING THE CONTRIBUTIONS OF THE BEHAVIORAL AND SOCIAL SCIENCES TO HEALTH

The Barbara and Jerome Grossman Symposium

Summary of the Institute of Medicine Symposium on Contributions of the Behavioral and Social Sciences to Health

Lisa F. Berkman, Ph.D., *editor*

Institute of Medicine

and

Division of Behavioral and Social Sciences and Education National Research Council

NATIONAL ACADEMY PRESS
Washington, D.C.

NATIONAL ACADEMY PRESS • 2101 Constitution Avenue, N.W. • Washington, DC 20418

NOTICE: The project that is the subject of this report was approved by the Governing Board of the National Research Council, whose members are drawn from the councils of the National Academy of Sciences, the National Academy of Engineering, and the Institute of Medicine. The members of the committee responsible for the report were chosen for their special competences and with regard for appropriate balance.

Support for this project was provided by a generous gift from Barbara and Jerome Grossman. The views presented in this report are those of the authors and are not necessarily those of the funding organizations.

International Standard Book Number 0-309-08442-3

Additional copies of this report are available for sale from the National Academy Press, 2101 Constitution Avenue, N.W., Box 285, Washington, DC 20055. Call (800) 624-6242 or (202) 334-3313 (in the Washington metropolitan area), or visit the NAP's home page at **www.nap.edu.** The full text of this report is available at **www.nap.edu.**

For more information about the Institute of Medicine, visit the IOM home page at **www.iom.edu.**

The serpent has been a symbol of long life, healing, and knowledge among almost all cultures and religions since the beginning of recorded history. The serpent adopted as a logotype by the Institute of Medicine is a relief carving from ancient Greece, now held by the Staatliche Museen in Berlin.

First Printing, July 2002
Second Printing, October 2002

THE NATIONAL ACADEMIES

National Academy of Sciences
National Academy of Engineering
Institute of Medicine
National Research Council

The **National Academy of Sciences** is a private, nonprofit, self-perpetuating society of distinguished scholars engaged in scientific and engineering research, dedicated to the furtherance of science and technology and to their use for the general welfare. Upon the authority of the charter granted to it by the Congress in 1863, the Academy has a mandate that requires it to advise the federal government on scientific and technical matters. Dr. Bruce M. Alberts is president of the National Academy of Sciences.

The **National Academy of Engineering** was established in 1964, under the charter of the National Academy of Sciences, as a parallel organization of outstanding engineers. It is autonomous in its administration and in the selection of its members, sharing with the National Academy of Sciences the responsibility for advising the federal government. The National Academy of Engineering also sponsors engineering programs aimed at meeting national needs, encourages education and research, and recognizes the superior achievements of engineers. Dr. Wm. A. Wulf is president of the National Academy of Engineering.

The **Institute of Medicine** was established in 1970 by the National Academy of Sciences to secure the services of eminent members of appropriate professions in the examination of policy matters pertaining to the health of the public. The Institute acts under the responsibility given to the National Academy of Sciences by its congressional charter to be an adviser to the federal government and, upon its own initiative, to identify issues of medical care, research, and education. Dr. Kenneth I. Shine is president of the Institute of Medicine.

The **National Research Council** was organized by the National Academy of Sciences in 1916 to associate the broad community of science and technology with the Academy's purposes of furthering knowledge and advising the federal government. Functioning in accordance with general policies determined by the Academy, the Council has become the principal operating agency of both the National Academy of Sciences and the National Academy of Engineering in providing services to the government, the public, and the scientific and engineering communities. The Council is administered jointly by both Academies and the Institute of Medicine. Dr. Bruce M. Alberts and Dr. Wm. A. Wulf are chairman and vice chairman, respectively, of the National Research Council.

Acknowledgments

The Institute of Medicine (IOM) would like to thank Barbara and Jerome Grossman for providing the funds to support this symposium. The symposium and publication of this report would not have been possible without their generous gift.

I would also like to thank each of the symposium speakers for their thoughtful, informative, and lively presentations. Their work has been and will continue to be instrumental in recognizing the importance of behavioral, social, economic, and environmental influences on health. I extend special appreciation to the symposium chair and report editor, Lisa F. Berkman, for keeping the lively discussions focused and moving forward throughout the day.

I would like to thank the following IOM and National Research Council (NRC) staff for their help in planning the symposium, drawing from their experience as staff officers on projects from which the symposium largely drew its content: Christine R. Hartel, Director of the Board on Behavioral, Cognitive, and Sensory Sciences, National Research Council; Terry C. Pellmar, Director, Board on Neuroscience and Behavioral Health; Brian D. Smedley, Study Director, Board on Health Sciences Policy, Institute of Medicine; and Alexandra K. Wigdor, Study Director, National Research Council.

I would also like to thank the following IOM staff for assisting in the logistics, planning, and execution of the symposium: Barbara D. Boyd,

Administrative Assistant, Institute of Medicine; Donna D. Duncan, Deputy Director, Office of Council and Membership Services, Institute of Medicine; Don Tiller, Senior Membership Assistant, Office of Council and Membership Services, Institute of Medicine; Hallie Wilfert, Manager of New Media, Institute of Medicine; and especially Leslie Baer, who stepped in at the last minute to do a terrific job of handling the meeting logistics. And a special thanks goes to Jennifer Otten, who took the lead in organizing this effort early on and who has played a continuing key role in this effort.

We also extend a special thanks to those who attended the symposium and continue to keep the dialogue alive.

Susanne A. Stoiber
Executive Officer
Institute of Medicine

Contents

Introduction

The importance of behavioral, social, economic, and environmental influences on health is increasingly recognized. Further, the relationships among genetic factors, social influences, and the physical environment are now of growing interest to the research, policy, public health, and clinical communities. As research in these areas yields new knowledge about these interactions, we are faced with the challenge of applying and translating that knowledge into practical applications or policy directions.

To advance this challenge, the Institute of Medicine (IOM) brought together experts and collaborators at a symposium in May 2001. The symposium featured five reports released in the last 12 months by the IOM and the Division of Behavioral and Social Sciences and Education (DBASSE). The reports were the starting point for assessing the status of behavioral and social science research relating to health, identifying where the greatest opportunities appear to lie in translating this research into clinical medicine, public health, and social policy; and recognizing the barriers that continue to impede significant progress in conducting and utilizing this field of research.

Symposium presenters were asked to look at these key questions and areas:

• What were the principal theoretical and practical problems encountered by the committees as they reviewed the relevant literature and what lessons can be drawn from their efforts that should guide those who fund and conduct research in this area?

- What are the key lessons to be drawn in terms of barriers to the conduct of this research and its application in medicine, public health, and public policy?
- What priorities emerged across the reports in terms of training needs, research opportunities, and translation into practice?
- What observations regarding the differences between behavioral and social sciences and the biological sciences might be useful to improve communication/collaboration?

This report is a proceedings of the symposium from these experts in the field. Topics covered include research design, training, infrastructure investments, grant making, etiology, interventions, and priority investments necessary to support rapid advances in the behavioral and social sciences.

Introduction to the Subject

Lisa F. Berkman
Harvard School of Public Health

Dr. Berkman opened her remarks by citing the six reports of the National Research Council and IOM that inspired this symposium. It is "stunning," she noted, that despite these reports' diversity—addressing children, aging, research priorities, training, health promotion, and interventions, among other topics—they all come to similar conclusions. They consistently say that social and behavioral conditions are major determinants of health and that this realization implies new ways to do science in order to improve the health of the public.

"Just as the natural sciences—biology and chemistry and even physics—have reorganized in terms of how they fundamentally teach and train people," said Dr. Berkman, "today we are building on the same kind of technological advancements and real achievements in the social sciences, and we are at a similar kind of crossroads."

The reports note the importance of a new concept, "population health," developed initially by Jeffrey Rose in 1992. He said that it was critical not only to ask why some individual patients get sick but also why this *population* has its own distribution of risk. He pointed out, for example, the differences in blood pressure patterns between London civil servants and Kenyan nomads; these distributions overlapped only slightly. Similarly, Dr. Berkman noted, virtually everyone in Finland today would have high serum cholesterol levels by Japanese standards (see Figure A).

A major population health issue in the United States, she said, is the epidemic of obesity among children. Three times as many kids in the 1990s

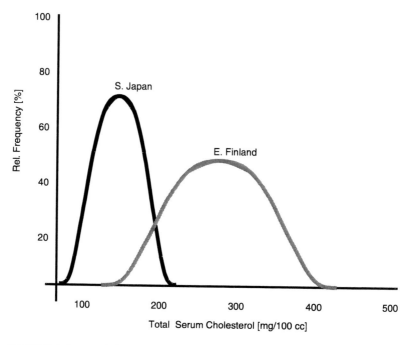

FIGURE A Serum cholesterol levels among populations in Japan and Finland.

were obese by standards set in the mid-1960s (see Figure B). More fundamentally, why has the mean weight of all children in the United States risen over the past 20 or 30 years, causing the percentage of kids in the tails of the distribution to be obese?

Another area of population health in which we have acquired a great deal of evidence, Dr. Berkman said, is social stratification and inequality. For example, between 1969 and 1998, mortality rates dropped dramatically among men in every socioeconomic group. But those in the lower socioeconomic status groups had higher mortality rates, and the gap between the highest and lowest groups actually grew.

There are dramatic health disparities in racial and ethnic groups as well. In Table 1, which shows life expectancy for white men and women and black men and women from 1950 to 1996, life expectancy is improving for everyone. But as black men enter the 21st century they have a life expectancy less than what white men enjoyed 46 years earlier. Black women do only a little better—their rates look like those of white women 36 years earlier.

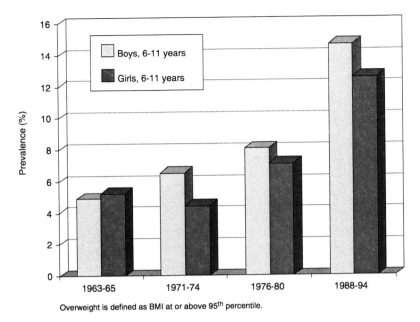

Overweight is defined as BMI at or above 95th percentile.

FIGURE B Obesity rates of children in the United States, 1963-1994.

Almost all the data suggest that the lower socioeconomic status of African Americans accounts for much, but not all, of this gradient, said Dr. Berkman. Some of the more important and innovative work in this area is identifying additional factors such as discrimination, which may lead to increased risk among certain racial and ethnic groups. "In a society where

TABLE 1 Life Expectancy at Birth for Blacks and Whites, 1950-1996

	Whites		Blacks	
	Men	Women	Men	Women
1950	66.5	72.2	58.9	62.7
1960	67.4	74.1	60.7	65.9
1970	68.0	75.6	60.0	68.3
1980	70.7	78.1	63.8	72.5
1990	72.7	79.4	64.5	73.6
1996	73.9	79.7	66.1	74.2

in the next 50 years we expect the minority to become the majority," she said, "we cannot afford to leave this issue unresolved."

Another area of research in which we have accumulated a great deal of evidence, Dr. Berkman said, is the importance of social relationships. Literally hundreds of studies now link social isolation to increased mortality, morbidity, and lower survival. And scores of studies identify attachment and caregiving as critical components of early childhood development.

Some of the most far-reaching and innovative research today has been on the "power of place." While research on neighborhoods has long been a tradition in social science, new findings indicate that work environments, school environments, cultures, and other social contexts also play important roles in determining individuals' health outcomes.

Given the consistency of such new findings in social science research, Dr. Berkman said, the six National Research Council and IOM reports exhibit several common, and critical, themes. Virtually all recognize that behaviors occur in a social context. If we could characterize earlier waves of behavioral interventions as individualistic—focusing on smoking cessation among individuals, for instance—the new wave of behavioral interventions is built on a recognition that where we live and work and who we talk to, and what kind of resources we have and where we buy our groceries, all shape our behavior.

Another critical theme of these reports is the importance of understanding multiple determinants of health, or multiple levels of influence, simultaneously. Social and economic policies at the upper levels, on down through institutions, neighborhoods, living conditions, social relationships, individual risk factors, genetic/constitutional factors, and pathophysiologic pathways, all contribute to individual and population health.

A third pervasive theme relates to life course and development; issues of cumulative disadvantage, latency, precursors of later resiliency, or disease risk are now central themes in many of these reports. However, this life-course perspective requires substantial new investments in the kinds of studies that we do, said Dr. Berkman. Longitudinal studies, whether they are cohorts starting from birth or young adulthood, or simply cohorts that take us through career trajectories in middle and older age, are profoundly needed in the United States.

The fourth theme of these reports, Dr. Berkman said, revolves around understanding the pathways that link the macro social structure to biologic mechanisms of disease causation. Harmful social experiences, and the cumulative wear and tear on the body through repeated activation of physiologic stress responses, affect a life's course.

Examples of such stress paradigms based on social conditions include the brain, where we see hippocampal shrinkage and memory loss; endocrine systems, where we see things like diabetes; cardiovascular systems that influence hypertension and coronary heart disease; and reproductive systems that may be related to low birth weight and ovarian function.

The persuasive evidence discussed in the reports has three basic implications for social and behavioral approaches to health, Dr. Berkman said. The first is that theories of disease causation that focus primarily on the individual should be complemented by the systematic patterning of risk across social contexts.

Second, we have new outcomes. No longer is it adequate to think only of mortality or disease-specific morbidity. We are dealing with health in a world where new issues of child development and aging—assessments of functioning from the standpoint of cognitive ability, optimal performance, and disability—are becoming increasingly important.

Third, we need new ways of intervening that integrate what we have recently learned. Ultimately, of course, our goal is not only to understand the determinants of health but to *improve* health. That means we will also need to develop new methods of training and new partnerships to improve the likelihood that interventions will be successful.

Thus, the next steps need to be really bold ones, Dr. Berkman said. They will require reconfigurations in funding opportunities across National Institute of Health (NIH) and foundations, for example, changes in educating the next generations of scientists and practitioners, and dissemination and press coverage that clearly get out the message that improvements in health depend in large part on changes in the social environment.

What We Know:
The Tantalizing Potential

ETIOLOGY, PART I

John Cacioppo
The University of Chicago

Dr. Cacioppo began his presentation on the concepts of social isolation and loneliness by pointing out what has been learned since Francis Crick articulated his central dogma of molecular biology some 30 years ago. Crick maintained that social and environmental influences on health were largely those codified in the DNA we've inherited from our ancestors of millennia past. These molecules direct the production of proteins in our bodies, which, among other things, underlie our behavior and sense of well-being.

But over the past few decades, Dr. Cacioppo said, we have learned that different environmental contexts produce different molecular-level reactions. The social environment not only operates in terms of genetic constitutions sculpted over thousands of years ago but also can affect the genetic processes of transcription and translation in the individual.

In a study conducted at Ohio State University, Dr. William Malarkey, Dr. Cacioppo, and colleagues showed that the amounts of growth hormone produced by B and T cells in the body were diminished in individuals who'd been exposed to chronic social stressors. The most likely means by

Isolation	Connectedness	Belongingness
• "I lack companionship" • "I feel left out" • "I feel isolated from others" • "I am unhappy being so withdrawn"	• "There are people to whom I feel close" • "There are people who really understand me" • "There are people to whom I can talk" • "There are people to whom I can turn"	• "I feel in tune with the people around me" • "I feel part of a group of friends" • "I have a lot in common with the people around me" • "My interests and ideas are not shared by those around me"

(N = 2,632 young adults who, developmentally speaking, were picking partners and establishing lifetime health habits)

FIGURE A Mechanisms that contribute to individual differences in loneliness.

which this was achieved, the authors posited, was through the down-regulatory influences of catecholamines and corticosteroids on lymphocytes.

One major factor responsible for chronic stress, as well as broad-based morbidity and mortality, is social isolation, though the mechanism by which it produces these adverse health effects has not been specified. In a series of studies of individual differences in loneliness—or the perception that one is socially isolated from others and bereft of meaningful human contact—the researchers tested various mechanisms that could contribute to this relationship (see Figure A). They studied over 2,600 young adults at Ohio State University and Stanford University because, developmentally speaking, they were selecting partners and establishing lifetime health habits. More recently, they have studied older adults whose physiological resilience could be expected to be diminished.

Dr. Cacioppo said that when we look at the psychological profiles of lonely individuals they "tend to be shy and possess poor social skills; report higher levels of stress, anxiety, and hostility; distrust other individuals and feel as if they are contributing more than their share to their relationships; be characterized by higher negative affectivity, pessimism, and negative reactivity; and respond to stressors less through active coping and seeking social support and more through withdrawal." In general, this profile is evident in personality and social inventories and in momentary reports using an experience sampling methodology to assess subjects' status during their normal daily life.

Although genetic studies of loneliness are rare, the extant data suggest that at least half the variance is attributable to environmental factors, Dr. Cacioppo said. It was not the case, for instance, that lonely individuals were characterized by lower levels of "social capital": lonely and nonlonely individuals did not differ in height, weight, body mass index, intelligence, physical attractiveness, family wealth, or any other sociodemographic variable they examined.

Additional evidence for the importance of environmental influences was provided by Dr. Cacioppo and Stanford's Dr. David Spiegel in a study in which they used hypnosis to manipulate the feelings of loneliness in a sample of adults at Stanford. They found that when these participants were led to feel lonely, they were characterized by the same psychological profile as the lonely individuals tested at Ohio State; when the Stanford participants were led to feel socially connected (not at all lonely), they were characterized by the same psychological profile as the socially connected individuals tested at Ohio State.

Poor health behaviors contribute to broad-based morbidity and mortality, so the health behaviors of lonely and nonlonely individuals were compared. Though results consistently show no differences, lonely individuals do report higher levels of stress, dysphoria, and anxiety. Individuals who are socially disconnected may be exposed to more stressors (direct effects), and when exposed to a stressor they may have less assistance to help them deal with it (stress buffering). Dr. Cacioppo and colleagues found additional evidence not only that lonely individuals were more stressed by daily hassles and events, but that restorative activities were less salubrious for the lonely than the nonlonely.

The quintessential restorative behavior is sleep. But in a sleep monitoring study, he said, "we found that lonely days invaded the nights. Lonely individuals showed poor sleep efficiency and more time awake after sleep onset," which cause the fatigue that one feels the next day. In both young and older adults, lonely individuals reported poorer sleep and more fatigue during the day than nonlonely adults.

Sleep disruptions, of course, can affect health. This was shown by Evan Carter and colleagues at the University of Chicago in a study published in *The Lancet* 2 years ago. After causing people to incur a sleep debt by depriving them of a great deal of sleep, the researchers found metabolic, neural, and hormonal effects that mimic those of aging.

Another important health-related parameter is blood pressure, which becomes elevated acutely, say, when giving a speech and becomes elevated chronically in many American adults as a function of age. Interestingly, the basal levels and stress-related elevations in blood pressure were found to be comparable for the lonely and nonlonely young adults, Dr. Cacioppo said, but important differences were found in the underlying cardiovascular activity. Lonely young adults were characterized by higher total peripheral resistance (the resistance to blood flow in the cardiovascular system), with normal blood pressures achieved through lower cardiac output than nonlonely adults. The same differences were found in the laboratory and in ambulatory recordings during the course of their normal day.

We wondered if, as in other systems that are chronically stressed over many years, we would start to see blood pressure rise in those individuals who had long been lonely, Dr. Cacioppo said. The answer appears to be yes. In a preliminary study of older adults, lonely participants were characterized by age-related increases in blood pressure, whereas the nonlonely older adults were spared this trend (see Figure B). Humans are social animals who benefit psychologically and physically from a sense of contact,

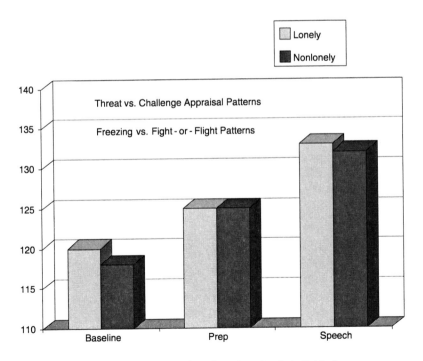

FIGURE B Systolic blood pressure of lonely and nonlonely individuals.

alliance, and community with others. When bereft of these feelings, every-day events appear more daunting, others appear more threatening, activities become more hopeless, and the nights become less restorative. Over time, such a mindset takes its toll on the body.

ETIOLOGY, PART II

Robert J. Sampson
The University of Chicago

Dr. Sampson began his presentation—on the association of health-related outcomes, especially lethal violence, with social context—by stating his thesis: we need to treat neighborhood and community contexts as important units of analysis in their own right, which in turn calls for new strategies that look well beyond the traditional approach of focusing largely on the individual. "Understanding the pathways to healthy and unhealthy communities," he said, "may provide opportunities for preventive intervention at lower costs than traditional strategies."

While there has been a long history in this country of differentiation across neighborhoods, Dr. Sampson observed, this pattern appears not to be receding but is in fact expanding. Recent research shows that the spatial separation of economic groups has increased and also that segregation by race/ethnicity remains very high and in some cases has increased as well. This intersection of socioeconomic context with race/ethnicity has hit African Americans and other minority groups especially hard. Regardless of individual or family differences, these groups disproportionately tend to live in areas of concentrated poverty.

Dr. Sampson noted that neighborhood inequality is definitely linked with well-being or the lack of it. "For at least a hundred years," he said, "research has shown that violence and other health-related outcomes are correlated especially with concentrated disadvantage. For example, research in the early 1920s showed that a number of health outcomes—not just crime and delinquency but things such as low birth weight, tuberculosis, physical abuse, and other factors detrimental to the well-being of individuals—were concentrated in certain areas and that these areas were disproportionately disadvantaged."

This general empirical finding continues to the present day, Dr. Sampson said, as illustrated by "ecological co-morbidity," or the spatial clustering of homicide, infant mortality, low birth weight, and other adverse health conditions.

The implication, he said, is that there are "hot spots" of poor health outcomes. For example, in a map he displayed of Chicago's distribution of homicides—literally, pinpoints of homicide events—from 1990 to 1996, there was distinct spatial clustering in particular neighborhoods (see Figure A). A similar map of the city that showed the distribution of another health outcome—low birth weight—revealed a very similar pattern (see Figure B). "If I didn't label these," he noted, "you'd probably have a hard time distinguishing between the two maps."

Homicides 1990-1996
(1 dot per homicide)

Low Birth Weight 1990-1996
(1 dot per 5 incidents)

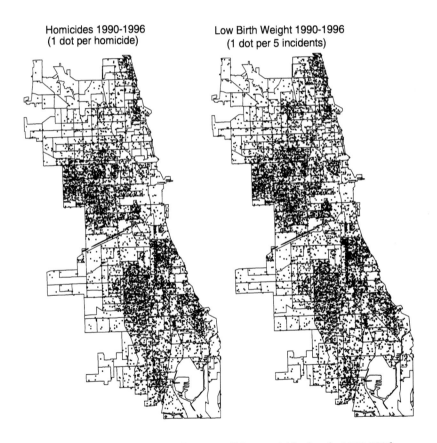

FIGURE A (left) Homicide distribution in Chicago neighborhoods, 1990-1996.

FIGURE B (right) Low birth weight distribution in Chicago Neighborhoods, 1990-1996.

Might this just be the result of vulnerable individuals being left behind in poor neighborhoods? Or perhaps of poor, unhealthy individuals migrating to certain communities? That is probably part of the story, Dr. Sampson said, but not the whole story. Neighborhood characteristics correlate with degrees of well-being even after individual attributes and risky behaviors are adjusted.

What are the underlying mechanisms? This is a very difficult issue to address, he said, but in a new generation of studies researchers are trying to systematically measure and elucidate neighborhood processes such as trust, social networks, informal social control, and the density and capacity of organizations—in other words, social structural features of the environment.

Dr. Sampson and colleagues are involved in one such interdisciplinary study, the Project on Human Development in Chicago Neighborhoods, that started in 1995. "It is essentially a 'life course,' or developmental, study not just of delinquent and violent behavior," he said, "but of achievement and various aspects of youth growing up. How are they doing well and how are they doing poorly? And how do outcomes—violence, for example—correlate with variations in neighborhood context?"

The study has focused on the "collective efficacy" of community members in achieving a common good, and it has looked at two features in particular: informal social control (the willingness and ability of adults in the neighborhood to be involved with local organizations and also to monitor and supervise the activities of children) and working trust among neighbors (not tight-knit social bonds, but rather a linkage of trust with shared expectations for action).

Basically, Dr. Sampson said, the project's research has shown that areas with higher degrees of collective efficacy have significantly lower rates of violence, all else being equal, and that this effect is observed regardless of the socioeconomic status of the community.

"However, I'm not here just to tell you that local collective features of neighborhoods matter," Dr. Sampson said. The social context of the larger urban environment also plays an important role that researchers often overlook. "Specifically, spatial proximity to disadvantage turns out to be one of the strongest predictors of homicide and some other health outcomes, regardless of the resources, racial composition, and socioeconomic status of individual neighborhoods."

He illustrated the concept of spatial vulnerability to risk with another map of Chicago (see Figure C). In addition to a clear connection between

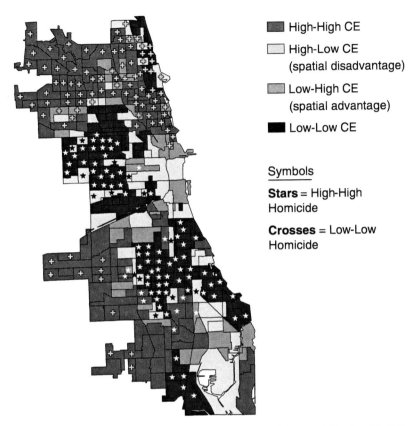

FIGURE C Spatial typology of collective efficacy (CE) with homicide "hot" and "cold" spots.

neighborhoods of low collective efficacy with hot spots and neighborhoods of high collective efficacy with cold spots, the map also revealed a different kind of risk: neighborhoods with high collective efficacy that are in close proximity to high-risk areas have very high homicide rates themselves. Conversely, "spatially advantaged" neighborhoods (which border low-risk areas) have low risks of homicide even when they are low in collective efficacy.

"So even though I would like to argue that neighborhood effects matter," Dr. Sampson said, "it is not just the neighborhoods but actually the embeddedness within the larger metropolitan context" that also matters.

Early Childhood Interventions: Theories of Change, Empirical Findings, and Research Priorities

INTERVENTIONS, PART I

Jack P. Shonkoff
Brandeis University

Dr. Shonkoff introduced his presentation as "a view from 30,000 feet"—an overview of the underlying science and reflections on the challenges facing the field. He began by outlining four characteristics of the current landscape of behavioral and social intervention:

• *Public skepticism.* "We face widespread questioning about whether we really know how to change behavior and influence developmental trajectories."

• *Expanding yet incomplete science.* "The rich and growing knowledge base that guides the design and implementation of behavioral and social interventions is conceptually strong but empirically uneven."

• *Demonstrated efficacy but inconsistent performance.* Model programs provide credible evidence that we have the capacity to intervene effectively, but successful demonstration projects typically "have different characteristics from the full range of interventions that are actually delivered when promising programs are brought to scale."

• *Complexity of successful service delivery.* "Interventions that work are rarely simple, inexpensive, or easy to implement."

Given the diversity of interventions that have been proposed and implemented, Dr. Shonkoff indicated that his remarks would focus on early childhood intervention as a prototype—to serve "as a heuristic model for thinking more broadly about how we might approach behavioral and social interventions across different ages and venues." Early childhood intervention, he said, is a useful model because it rests on a sound theoretical framework, builds on a strong experimental base, and provides promising foundations for a life-span strategy because of its prevention orientation.

Effective interventions in the early childhood years have a number of distinguishing features, Dr. Shonkoff said. The first is the importance of an individualized approach linked to specific objectives. In contrast, programs that are built on a one-size-fits-all model and guided by broad generic goals are relatively ineffective.

A second feature of successful programs is the high quality of their implementation. Central to this success is a well-designed intervention strategy, appropriate staff training, and careful monitoring of service delivery over time.

A third feature of effective interventions in the early childhood period is the quality of the relationships that are built between the people who provide the service and those who receive it. The positive "effects of relationships on relationships" may be at the heart of what makes early childhood interventions work, Dr. Shonkoff said. "That is to say, the provider-parent relationship influences the parent-child relationship, which, in turn, can result in positive outcomes for both the child and the parents."

A fourth feature—that early childhood intervention be family centered, community based, and coordinated—"is embedded in a strong theoretical framework," Dr. Shonkoff said, "but has not been sufficiently validated empirically." For example, the widespread belief that programs are more effective when delivered through parents rather than focused directly on children may or may not be true in all circumstances, as we do not have sufficient experimental data on this dimension of service delivery. This "is an important issue because high levels of parent involvement in early childhood programs are more difficult to achieve than they were when fewer mothers were in the workforce."

The last feature of effective interventions relates to the critical dimensions of program timing, intensity, and duration. Here again, "the field is replete with strong opinions," Dr. Shonkoff said, but "the empirical knowledge base is thin." We do have persuasive indications about the benefits of earlier initiation and longer duration of services—for example, demonstration programs for children in poverty that have been the most effective started either prenatally or in early infancy and extended up through school. "But answers to questions about cutoff points for 'early' versus 'late,' and hard data on intensity and frequency of specific service components, await further study."

Dr. Shonkoff then proceeded to discuss some of the "persistent challenges" that remain to be addressed by the early childhood intervention field. These include:

• *Expanding access and participation.* "Many young children who have the greatest need for services often don't get them," he said, "either because the programs don't reach out effectively into communities with the most vulnerable populations or because families choose not to participate."

• *Ensuring greater quality control, particularly when bringing successful models to scale.* "We have a problematic track record," Dr. Shonkoff said, "of taking interventions that have been demonstrated to be effective in model settings, and then trying to do them 'on the cheap' by serving larger numbers of children with fewer staff who are trained less well and compensated more poorly."

• *Defining and achieving "cultural competence."* One of the important contexts in which young children develop is the culture of the family and of the community in which they live. Consequently, the call for early childhood intervention services that are culturally competent has become a growing political mandate. Dr. Shonkoff noted, however, that "we have very little hard knowledge" about this compelling and complex issue. "How we define cultural competence, how we teach it, and how we embed it in all of our intervention programs is an emerging area of scientific inquiry."

• *Identifying and responding to the special needs of distinctive subgroups.* Most traditional models of early childhood intervention are not well designed to address significant family problems that can have major adverse impacts on child well-being. "Family violence, substance abuse, and parental mental illness, particularly maternal depression, are three common examples," Dr. Shonkoff said. The challenge is to reconcile the core competencies that must be available within all early childhood programs with the specialized professional expertise that may be required to address a wide variety of serious family needs.

• *Reducing fragmentation and strengthening the service infrastructure.* "The world of early childhood programs is characterized by highly fragmented policies and service systems that have been developed independently to address the needs of children living in poverty, children with disabilities, children who have been abused or neglected, and children who need generic care and early education. Consequently, we have many children whose complex needs are addressed separately by multiple service streams, with limited integration across systems," Dr. Shonkoff said. Though dealing with that fragmentation is essentially a political issue, the scientific community can help by articulating the unified knowledge base that cuts across the multiple service systems.

• *Assessing costs and making choices among alternative investments.* The broad-based and multifaceted system of early childhood intervention has not had a tradition of looking carefully at costs and benefits or measuring cost effectiveness. Dr. Shonkoff urged that such concerns be given considerably more attention, particularly when assessing the impacts of complex interventions with multiple components.

Dr. Shonkoff concluded his presentation by calling for a "dramatic rethinking about the interactions among the science, the policy, and the practice" of behavioral and social interventions across the life span, using early-childhood intervention as a model. Three issues were highlighted.

First, he said, is the need to reconcile traditional service strategies with the economic and social realities of contemporary family life. Second is the need to improve the availability, training, and compensation of service providers in the field. Finally, Dr. Shonkoff underscored "the need to change the highly politicized context in which intervention programs are evaluated, which results in a high-stakes environment that undermines honest attempts to improve quality." He noted that evaluators and service providers often underplay evidence of ineffective services and overstate the extent to which programs do work. Alternatively, Dr. Shonkoff called for "a more constructive culture of intervention research that asks hard questions about what is working, disseminates evidence of effective services and promotes their implementation, shines an equally bright light on programs that are not working, and goes 'back to the drawing board' to generate new approaches to behaviors that are more resistant to change."

INTERVENTIONS, PART II

Margaret Chesney
University of California, San Francisco

Dr. Chesney began her presentation by noting some of the progress over the past few decades in improving individuals' health behaviors. Adult smoking prevalence, for example, has decreased by about 40 percent since the Surgeon General's report of 1964. And behavioral interventions in studies over the last 25 years have increased average weight loss by 75 percent and physical activity frequency by up to 25 percent.

Still, she noted, much remains to be done. Over 24 percent of adults in the United States still smoke. A majority of adult Americans—some 60 percent—are now considered overweight, and 18 percent of the adult population is deemed obese. In addition, there is evidence of a new epidemic of obesity among youth. Meanwhile, despite all the attention to exercise, only 24 percent of the U.S. population regularly engages in light-to-moderate activity.

So on balance, Dr. Chesney said, we know that "behavioral interventions can lead to improvements in health, but that these improvements need to be maintained over time and reach all ethnic, racial, social class, and gender groups. They also need to be extended to the population at large across our neighborhoods."

Dr. Chesney said she is optimistic that these challenges can be met, and the remainder of her talk largely addressed her four basic reasons: The first reason is that an important shift in the basic nature of interventions has been occurring and will likely last. We are shifting from a treatment model—which has addressed unhealthy behaviors the way medicine approaches infections, as pathogens responsive to short-term therapy or surgical intervention—to "a model that recognizes that behavior is controlled by complex social contingencies."

If we want to change peoples' diets, their level of physical activity, or other lifestyle factors, Dr. Chesney said, "It is not like a bacterial infection, for which one could administer five sessions of health counseling like an antibiotic and expect that the unhealthy dietary habits or the physical inactivity would be 'cured.' Changing behavior is more like managing diabetes; it requires monitoring and care over time."

The second reason for optimism, she said, is "the increasing diversity of interventions and approaches that are being tested and implemented. In particular, interventions are increasingly being developed to respond to the needs of different community groups. Interventions are targeting higher-risk populations, tailored to individuals or to groups, and designed in ways that are more culturally appropriate."

The third and perhaps most compelling reason for optimism, discussed and embedded in the six National Research Council and Institute of Medicine (IOM) reports, is the importance of the social context in which the behavior occurs.

This understanding is reflected, Dr. Chesney said, in the social ecology model developed by Daniel Stokols of the University of California, Irvine. An individual's behavior, rather than being seen as an isolated event and the responsibility of the individual alone, is considered to be influenced by or the result of a number of factors: intrapersonal factors (including motivation, skills, attitudes); interpersonal factors (social networks, norms, the influence of one's neighborhood); the institutions and organizations in which the person works or goes to school; and the public policies that broadly influence his or her life.

Thus, as Tracy Orleans of the Robert Wood Johnson Foundation put it, "we need to expand the targets of successful interventions beyond the individual to the powerful social contexts in which they live." Interventions may be focused at multiple levels to achieve change, including what John B. McKinlay of the New England Research Institutes has called the "downstream" level (individualized approaches and interventions), the "midstream" level (interventions at homes, work sites, schools, and churches), and the "upstream" level (efforts to change social policies through media and legislation that reward health).

The impressive achievements in tobacco control, for example, may be attributed to the simultaneous efforts at each of these levels. Over the past decades, "downstream" interventions consisting of individual counseling and group smoking cessation programs have improved quit rates. At the same time, "midstream" interventions worked to prevent smoking initiation and to encourage smoking cessation with school-based, work site, and community programs. Tobacco control efforts also illustrate the impact of "upstream" interventions, with policy-level approaches such as the Food and Drug Administration (FDA) regulations designed to reduce the availability and impact of tobacco marketing aimed at youth.

Tobacco control has moved even farther upstream. It became apparent that the reliance of farmers in the southeastern United States on tobacco crops created pressure to maintain a tobacco market. Dr. Chesney described efforts to help tobacco farmers transition to new enterprises, new commodities, and new crops as "very upstream" interventions. In these efforts, it is especially critical to work not only with the farmers themselves but with their neighborhoods, communities, and churches—the social contexts in which they live—which for centuries have supported and have been supported by the tobacco crop.

Dr. Chesney's fourth and most important reason for optimism, she said, is that such multilevel interventions, which address risk behaviors in the social context that supports them, are beginning to show effects. She cited the Treatwell 5-A-Day Study, carried out by Glorian Sorenson and her colleagues at the Dana-Farber Cancer Institute, as an example. Community health centers in the Northeast were randomly assigned to one of three treatment arms: some community health centers had only a work-site intervention; others had a work-site-plus-family intervention; and a third group of centers, which had only a minimal intervention, served as the control.

In the first group, people in participating community health centers received the Treatwell 5-A-Day series of 10 interventions aimed at improving diet in general and increasing their intake of fruits and vegetables in particular, and they were exposed to annual campaigns in nutrition education. In addition, health center staff actively worked with them to make changes in their work site that would increase the availability of healthy foods in snack rooms, vending machines, and throughout the work setting. "They were directly impacting the social environment in which people lived to change the way that they ate," Dr. Chesney said.

Community health centers assigned to a work-site-plus-family intervention did all of the above but also went one step farther. They provided a five-session "Fit in 5" program in which families could learn at home, along with newsletters and other follow-up incentives, events, and materials designed to motivate the family to change its dietary habits.

At the end of this 19-month program, the groups that received the work site and family interventions showed significantly greater increases in fruit and vegetable intake than the control group (which received only a modest amount of dietary information). Most impressively, the increase in the work-site-plus-family intervention group was almost three times that of the group exposed to work site interventions alone (see Figure A).

The focus of this talk, Dr. Chesney said, was the contribution of behavioral interventions to health promotion and disease prevention. But she

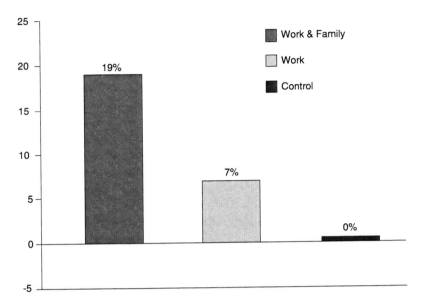

FIGURE A Treatwell 5-A-Day study in fruit and vegetable intake.

also wanted to briefly mention *psychosocial* interventions, such as those aiming to reduce stress, depression, depressed mood, and social isolation.

"Here we do have growing evidence that psychosocial interventions, which target coping skills and provide social support, can contribute to treatment, particularly in chronic disease management," she said. "These interventions, which are typically individual- and group-based, also need now to move from the downstream level to midstream and upstream . . . so that they reach more diverse groups and populations across our entire nation." We need a stronger science base there as well, she added.

Dr. Chesney concluded by noting that the time has come "for us to design, to test, and to implement behavioral and social interventions to improve health across the life span, beginning with the very young, and including the growing numbers of the oldest old, and to extend these efforts to the diverse groups that populate our communities."

This will require an ambitious but attainable partnership of public health officials, researchers, and community members. Her hope, she said, is that "when I come here in 2010 and we talk about . . . the objectives of Healthy People 2010, we can say that we have actually hit 100 percent" of those objectives.

Why Exploiting This Knowledge Will Be Essential to Achieving Health Improvements in the 21st Century

Raynard S. Kington
National Institutes of Health

Dr. Kington began his presentation by noting that projections from 1990 to the year 2050 show a steady decrease in the percentage of the U.S. population that is white and substantial increases in minority populations, particularly Hispanic and Asian. Hispanics, he said, will likely surpass African Americans as the country's largest minority group well before the middle of this century.

"The reason why [such] changes in composition of the population are potentially important," Dr. Kington said, "is because there are large differences in health outcomes across these subgroups." He illustrated these differences. Recent data (covering 1980-1996) show much higher mortality for African Americans than for any other group (the African American mortality rate is about 50 percent higher than that of whites); there is a clustering of mortality rates among non-Hispanic whites, American Indians, and Alaska Natives; and the rates are substantially lower for Hispanics and Asians (see Figure A).

Similarly, 1995 data show that infants born of African American mothers suffer more than twice the mortality rates as those of Hispanics and non-Hispanic whites (which have virtually the same infant mortality rates), and the rates among Asian and Pacific Islanders are yet lower (see Figure B).

"But simplistic slides like that really hide a substantial amount of heterogeneity within the large groups, in particular the Hispanic groups and the Asian American groups," Dr. Kington said. For example, infant mortal-

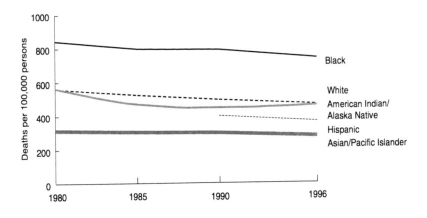

FIGURE A Mortality rates by race, 1980-1996.

ity rates for Puerto Ricans are substantially higher than those of Mexicans, Cubans, and Hispanics from Central and South America (see Figure C).

The reason for large differences in health outcomes among racial and ethnic groups in the United States, he said, "is the list of usual suspects: socioeconomic status, culture/acculturation, health risk behaviors, psycho-

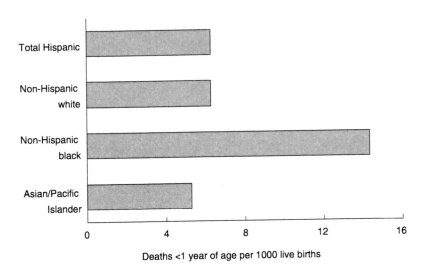

FIGURE B Infant mortality rates by race, 1995.

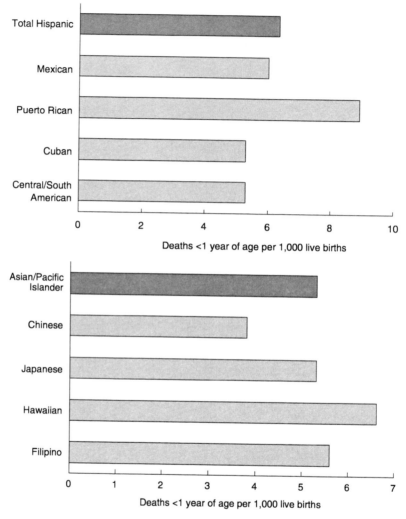

FIGURE C Infant mortality rates by Hispanic subgroup and Asian/Pacific Islander subgroup, 1995.

social factors, health care, biologic genetic factors, and environmental and occupational exposures." His talk expanded on the first two.

Some of the differences in health outcomes can be largely accounted for by socioeconomic status, Dr. Kington said. For example, "when we just stratify by educational attainment, we see that the mortality rates for those who have at least some college education is substantially lower than for those who have either just a high school education or have less than a high school education. [The latter group has] almost three times the mortality rate of those who have at least some college." Similarly, with respect to income, while all groups' wages increased substantially through the late 1960s and early 1970s, there has been a large spread since then in the changes in wages according to percentile in the population—with those at the lowest percentile having *decreases*—as well as a widening gap between the incomes of the highest and the lowest.

"The reason why this is relevant for the population at large and particularly relevant for minority populations," Dr. Kington said, "is because minority populations are overrepresented along that lowest line at the bottom end of the income structure." For example, over 50 percent of African American and Hispanic children live in households below 150 percent of the poverty line for income. "This is particularly relevant in light of the growing evidence suggesting that early life exposures and health factors set individuals on trajectories that will affect their health status for the rest of their lives."

Another reason for large differences in health outcomes among racial and ethnic groups in the United States, Dr. Kington said, is believed to be acculturation. And "the single most important finding in this area is that an increasing number of studies have described health behaviors and health outcomes among immigrant populations as *worsening* with acculturation."

For example, across a wide range of groups—including non-Hispanic whites, blacks, Asian subgroups, and Hispanic subgroups—all of the foreign-born populations have lower infant mortality rates than their U.S.-born counterparts. Dr. Kington declined to speculate on the reasons for this counterintuitive though "remarkably persistent finding." But he noted that the "behavioral and social sciences have the potential to address some of the most pressing health problems that the country is facing—particularly those problems related to differences in health status across racial and ethnic groups and across groups as stratified by socioeconomic status."

High-priority areas in which the behavioral and social sciences are especially well poised to make substantial contributions, he said, include:

• reducing the infant mortality rate, especially among poor women—and poor black women in particular;

- preventing deterioration of health status and health behaviors with acculturation of the growing immigrant population;
- intervening in the early years of life to prevent the trajectories of health status that seem to be determined by social factors during that period;
- developing appropriate interventions to promote healthier lifestyles among the growing Hispanic, Asian, and African American communities; and
- informing the development of nonhealth interventions to promote improved health status.

Dr. Kington closed by citing his favorite quote from Martin Luther King's *Letter from a Birmingham Jail*: "Human progress never rolls in on wheels of inevitability."

"Clearly, in order for these changes to occur, we have to *make* them occur," Dr. Kington said. "We have to think of ways to facilitate the translation of the scientific findings that we have in the behavioral and social sciences into real interventions that work in real populations and improve the health status of real people."

Refocus

Lisa F. Berkman
Harvard School of Public Health

To characterize the morning's presentations, Dr. Berkman pointed out some of the things they shared, such as strong science. "A decade ago, we would have said that [ours] is a weaker science, with *hints* at important things but not really reporting very conclusive findings."

When you look back at the results that John Cacioppo and Robert Sampson presented, however, you see really incredible strength emerging, she said. You also see, with regard to the intervention issues laid out by Jack Shonkoff and Margaret Chesney, a great deal of progress. "On a small scale and in lots of ways," Dr. Berkman said, "we know a lot about what we are doing, though scaling up [presents problems] of enormous magnitude."

Another point that the morning's presentations shared, she said, is that our society is undergoing rapid and often fundamental changes, most of them demographic. For example, the community hyper-segregation mentioned in Dr. Sampson's talk—both in terms of racial and ethnic segregation as well as socioeconomic segregation—is really quite a new phenomenon. "In some ways, we are not talking about the same thing just getting a little bit worse," she said. We are talking about something dramatically changing, and it has wide-ranging implications for what we are going to do."

Similarly, speakers discussed a growing inequality—particularly the spread over time in wages for different kinds of groups—that has "quite dramatic" implications, Dr. Berkman said. And also "very staggering" was Raynard Kington's point about acculturation. "Considering the magnitude

29

of patterns of migration coming into the United States, we could be in for some very important surprises," she said. "People could be doing very well, and then suddenly take a big turn for the worse" in succeeding generations.

Dr. Berkman said she was particularly taken with Jack Shonkoff's comment about the need for realistic social models when designing early-childhood interventions. "He didn't say this, but I'll say it—we can't pretend that women are at home all the time and don't work," she said. If you assume "that families look the way they did in the 1950s, you are in for a very rude awakening." Dr. Berkman called these speakers' points "important wake-up calls" that give us no choice but to change. "They really call upon us to think about things in a different way."

Thus the symposium will focus this afternoon on "a new way of doing business in order to make future progress in this area," she said. That will involve some struggles, beginning with the challenges of doing multidisciplinary work. But that is to be expected, as Dr. Kington so aptly reminded the audience with his quote of Martin Luther King.

Research to Understand the Mechanisms Through Which Social and Behavioral Factors Influence Health

Bruce S. McEwen
The Rockefeller University

"What is a biologist doing in a meeting on social and behavioral science?" Dr. McEwen rhetorically asked. Two good reasons, he said: "Biology underlies individual and social behavior; and individual behavior and the social environment exert powerful effects on health."

To illustrate the "gradients of health across the range of socioeconomic status," he showed a graph that plotted a number of disorders—osteoporosis, chronic disease, hypertension, and cervical cancer—as a function of socioeconomic status, from its highest to lowest levels (see Figure A). Morbidity rates climbed sharply and steadily as socioeconomic status decreased.

The brain plays a central role here by interpreting and responding to environmental factors—work, neighborhood, relationships, family, major life events, trauma, and abuse—that influence people in every walk of life, Dr. McEwen said. As a neurobiologist, he is particularly interested in studying two brain areas—the amygdala, which has to do with fear and strong emotions; and the hippocampus, which affects spatial, declarative, episodic, and contextual memory. "We all know that we remember best the things that are connected to strong emotions, either positive or negative; the amygdala provides that emotional jolt," he said. "The hippocampus provides the contextual memory—that is, where we were and what we were doing."

These two brain areas regulate hypothalamic output to the autonomic nervous system and to the neuroendocrine system, which promote adaptation. "And we [use] the term 'allostasis,' which literally means maintaining

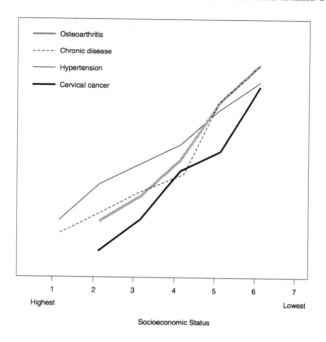

FIGURE A Morbidity rates by socioeconomic status level.

stability or homeostasis through active change, to refer to this process of adaptation," Dr. McEwen said. If allostatic mechanisms remain on too long or are overused, they increase the "allostatic load," a measure of the physiologic cost to different systems in the body from repeated burdens in one's life.

Other contributions of biology to psychosocial studies include providing information on the biological basis of resilience, often referred to as "positive health"; on the early warning signs for the risk of disease, called "predisease pathways"; and of course on the human genetic code, and the expression of its genes, now in the process of being deciphered.

Biologists can provide information on the interactions between the body's systems, Dr. McEwen noted. For example, diabetes, renal disease, and depression were the subjects of a workshop earlier this year at the National Institutes of Health. Other problems that need study across systems, he said, include cognitive disability in chronic pain and chronic fatigue; the consequences of sleep deprivation (which involve changes in immune function, metabolism, and cognition); and the wide-ranging results of anxiety disorder, which affects cardiovascular systems, metabolic systems, and immune systems.

Research using animal models has made many important contributions, Dr. McEwen said. Studies on monkeys, for example, "have taught us a lot about dominance and subordination and the rate of atherosclerosis and also suppression of immune function and the development of obesity." Studies on rats show that quality of maternal care can result in lifelong patterns of increased or decreased anxiety states.

"Genes, early life events, experiences (some of which we refer to as stress), lifestyle, and individual behavior," he said, are the important "players" here. They result in the cumulative wear and tear that is the cost of adaptation, referred to earlier as allostatic load, which "implies there are predisease pathways that we need to better understand in order to perform interventions before there is a real disease."

The mechanisms, or "mediators," involved in handling allostatic load include the autonomic nervous system, the neuroendocrine system, and the immune system, Dr. McEwen said. But while mediators in the short run have protective effects, in the long run they can exacerbate disease.

The best-known examples, he said, include cardiovascular disease, "where the acute activation of the sympathetic nervous system is involved in an animal fleeing from a predator and increasing its heart rate and also mobilizing energy stores. But chronic activation of the same system [can] accelerate atherosclerosis, particularly in a dominant animal vying for position in an unstable dominance hierarchy." From metabolism, he added, "we know very well that the hormones cortisol and catecholamines are involved in mobilizing and replenishing energy stores. But these same hormones participate in the development of insulin resistance and obesity and increased risk for cardiovascular disease."

To apply some of this information, the University of California at Los Angeles (UCLA)'s Theresa Seeman—like Dr. McEwen, a researcher in the MacArthur Network—and colleagues collected urinary cortisol and catecholamines samples, among others, in a group of subjects participating in the MacArthur Successful Aging Study. The researchers also devised a simple scoring system that correlated the measurements of these samples with the degree of allostatic load—the lower, the better. In that way, Dr. McEwen said, Seeman was able "to predict decline in both physical and cognitive function [and] predict new cardiovascular disease over two and a half years. . . . She also found a higher score with lower income, a higher score with lower education, and a lower score with higher social ties."

Other work, by Carol Ryff, Burton Singer, and colleagues in the Wisconsin Longitudinal Study, has found that the allostatic load in adulthood—among subjects in their 50s and 60s—is related to critical relationships. If subjects had at least one caring parent when growing up and a good-quality relationship with a spouse, this was defined as a positive pathway. Having uncaring or abusive parents when growing up, and/or a poor relationship with a spouse in adulthood, is a negative pathway. "The people with negative pathways, both men and women, had substantially higher allostatic load scores than people who had the more positive pathways," Dr. McEwen said (see Figure B).

Future work, Dr. McEwen said, should draw on additional "primary mediators," such as cytokines, anabolic hormones, and antioxidants, that have effects on many systems and are easy to measure. Similarly, we need "secondary outcomes," like cholesterol, bone marrow density, and atrophy of brain structures like the hippocampus and prefrontal cortex, to serve as "functional markers" of immune, cardiovascular, and cognitive function.

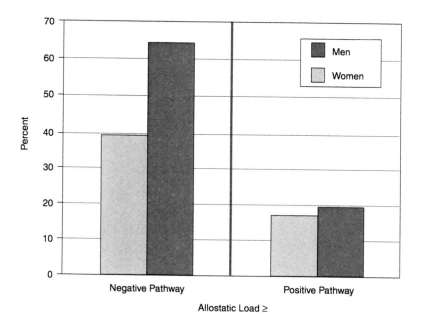

FIGURE B Relationship profiles and allostatic load.

These predisease markers can then "be used and measured longitudinally to find interventions that are effective in altering the course toward later disease," he said. "The well-accepted model of preventing atherosclerosis in heart disease by exercise and lowering cholesterol needs to be expanded to other disorders."

We also would benefit from more cross-system studies, he said. "We need to maintain a life-course perspective and think about early life events and their effects on later life outcomes—not just in aging, but in midlife. [We should] be particularly interested in understanding gene-environment interactions now that we understand more about the fact that it is not nature or nurture, but nature *interacting* with nurture. And of course, [we must] include behavioral and social environment as important factors in causing changes in biology."

He noted that "it is somewhat ironic that the National Institutes of Health primarily studies disease, not the factors of positive health and resilience." This highlights the biggest and most fundamental challenge, Dr. McEwen said, which is to promote "the establishment of working groups that will give scientists time to get acquainted with each other, learn about each other's disciplines, and plan interdisciplinary studies."

Investments in Longitudinal Surveys, Databases, Advanced Statistical Research, and Computation Technology

Robert M. Hauser
University of Wisconsin

Dr. Hauser introduced his presentation as a "survey of surveys"—in particular, of major longitudinal surveys. First he described their features:

- They represent real populations, either regional or national.
- The number of cases is large, usually several thousand households or persons.
- Their content covers a wide window in time, preferably decades rather than years.
- They measure key variables in multiple content domains and thus invite multidisciplinary research.
- The same variables are measured repeatedly across time, or retrospective histories are obtained.

The remainder of this "survey of [major longitudinal] surveys" would proceed in the following order: the big ones, epidemiological panel studies, some small (but good) ones, past or lost ones, offshore properties, and future prospects.

THE BIG ONES

These include the Health and Retirement Survey, the Longitudinal Studies of Aging, the National Long-Term Care Survey, the National Survey of Families and Households, Americans' Changing Lives, the Panel Study of Income Dynamics, and the Wisconsin Longitudinal Study.

The *Health and Retirement Survey* is a prospective study, now including more than 20,000 adults. It started in 1992-1993, and it has basically become a continuous longitudinal survey of all cohorts in the United States over the age of 50. "This is just a terrific vehicle; it is the Cadillac of such surveys," Dr. Hauser said. "It doesn't attempt to do everything for everybody. There is a specific emphasis on policies affecting retirement, health insurance, savings, and economic well-being." Some of its topics include health, disability and cognition, retirement plans, a variety of attitudes and preferences, family structure and transfers, employment status, job history and requirements, housing, income and net worth, health insurance, and pension plans.

The *Longitudinal Studies of Aging* were two six-year panel studies—the first in 1984, the second in 1994, with each followed biennially through four waves. The samples were drawn from the National Health Interview Survey, Dr. Hauser said, and the two studies ascertain a long list of self-reported social and health conditions such as housing characteristics, family structure and living arrangements, relationships and social contracts, and use of community services.

The *National Long-Term Care Survey* has gone through five panels from the early 1980s through 1999. Though it addresses the entire aged population—data are drawn from Medicare records—there is a focus on the functionally impaired. It provides very good data on trends in disability and mortality, he said.

The *National Survey of Families and Households,* which began in 1987-1988 and is now entering its third wave, "has really reinvented the sociology of the family in the United States," Dr. Hauser said. The design study focuses on relationships between parents and children, spouses and ex-spouses, ex-spouses and children, cohabitors—"all of these possible role relationships that now exist in abundance among American families."

Americans' Changing Lives, another broad-based population survey that started with 3,600 cases in 1986, has gone through three waves and is about to enter its fourth. It focuses on "productive" social relationships and cross-cultural variations within them, as well as on stressful events, chronic strains, and their effects on health functioning and productive activity. This survey has a substantial oversample of black Americans, Dr. Hauser said, and a lot of the activity focuses on comparisons between blacks and whites.

The *Panel Study of Income Dynamics* is an annual household survey that started with a poverty focus in 1968 and included 5,000 families. It has grown in size because "everybody gets followed, wherever they go, as they leave the original households and form new households," Dr. Hauser said. Its content now involves a central focus on demographic and economic stability and change, but there are numerous supplements—for example, the National Institute on Aging has supported supplements on health, health expenditures, housing, savings, pensions, and retirement.

The *Wisconsin Longitudinal Study* started out in 1957 with 10,317 high school graduates who were followed in 1964, 1975, 1992, and "we hope, again soon," Dr. Hauser said. The study has mostly focused on education, careers, and families and "is very rich in measures obtained in adolescence—including IQ, educational and occupational aspirations, social background, and other kinds of social influences" (such as school characteristics). Since 1992, he noted, "we have been picking up health, wealth, and well-being."

EPIDEMIOLOGICAL PANEL STUDIES

Dr. Hauser mentioned two well-known examples: the Alameda County Health and Ways of Living Study, "which followed a very nice long study of a community sample from the mid-1960s to the mid-1990s," and the Established Populations for Epidemiologic Studies of the Elderly, which covered 1981-1993.

SOME SMALL (BUT GOOD) ONES

The Terman study "is in some sense a model for everything that follows and in other ways absolutely horrible," Dr. Hauser said. "They selected all of the participants in the study on the basis of the value of the one variable that they thought was important—mental ability. Then the study went forward from there. But they followed these people all the way—from childhood to middle childhood to maturity and beyond—and they did that very well indeed."

Another three very small studies tend to get grouped together, he said, because their data are often analyzed together: the Berkeley Growth Study, the Berkeley Guidance Study, and the Oakland Growth Study. Then there is the Nun Study—a small survey of a select group. "Yet it has so far produced at least two absolutely astonishing and important findings," Dr. Hauser said, "because the window of observation is so long—from late adolescence through senescence and death—and because the quality of measurement is extraordinary across that span and because the content spans the social, the psychological, and the biological. That is where the payoff is, and what we have to do is get that kind of payoff from general population studies." Finally, the MacArthur studies of successful aging, also relatively small, "have given us some wonderful and provocative findings," he said, as mentioned earlier in this symposium.

PAST OR LOST ONES

Two examples are the now-defunct Project Talent—"a study of adolescents in 1960 that originally had some 400,000 high school kids enrolled, and quite possibly the worst longitudinal study ever conducted," Dr. Hauser said, and the National Longitudinal Studies, which focused "on labor market experience and are pretty much in the past." On the other hand, a historical reconstruction survey by the University of Chicago's Robert Fogel and collaborators—based on records of men who were in the Union Army during the Civil War—is "amazingly wonderful"—an "important historical record that . . . connects the medical and the social."

OFFSHORE PROPERTIES

"The British have done this better than anybody else," Dr. Hauser said, "with birth cohorts of 1946, 1958, and 1970 that cover all of the right stuff." Other nations—Germany and Australia, for example—have done excellent work as well. And the Indonesian and Malaysian Family Life Surveys, each spanning about a dozen years, "show that you can do very high-quality longitudinal research, again combining the social and the biomedical, in places where we wouldn't think of it as being so easy to do that kind of work."

FUTURE PROSPECTS

"The real point here is that we have to start thinking now about very young people who, with any luck at all, are going to get to be old," Dr. Hauser said. He referred to several school-based national cohort studies that ought to be followed up. Similarly with regard to household-based national cohort studies—such as the National Longitudinal Study of Youth, from 1979, which "has been immensely successful throughout its life." In the new panel of 1997, he said, "people should be thinking now about what we would like to know [about those kids] 50 or 60 or even 70 years from now."

STRENGTHS AND WEAKNESSES

"The real strength of longitudinal studies," Hauser said, "is that they give you 'the big picture,' a true description of the life course in real populations." Moreover, he added, "they permit quantitative analysis of social, economic, psychological, and biological processes as they occur. Studies that are relational or multilevel in design—e.g., including spouses, siblings, schools, employers, and localities—can provide important findings about social interaction and environmental or contextual influences on the life course." A final advantage, he said, is that, "because of the large number of participants in such studies, it is sometimes possible to study what happens in rare or narrowly defined populations—e.g., parents who have experienced the death or mental illness of a child."

"Most of the studies that I have described to you are of short duration—at least are *still* of short duration," Dr. Hauser added. "So we have to have the commitment to keep them going. We can't get tired of them any time too soon."

He also pointed out some of the challenges inherent in such studies. Many "are short on bioindicators. . . . With most of them, the only bioindicator we have is death." Also, "rich as they are, they can't really help us to solve questions of the difference between causation and correlation." They are expensive—the Health and Retirement Survey alone now costs about $9 million a year. There are real problems of coverage; many of these studies "have very serious problems of attrition. And some of them actually have rather poor coverage on the first round."

In the final phase of his talk, Dr. Hauser enumerated the goals for a system of longitudinal studies as follows:

• *Multidisciplinary.* "We need multidisciplinary integration in design, measurement, and analysis."
• *Multiplicity.* "We shouldn't put all of our eggs in one basket."
• *Overlap and complementarity.* We need "different studies specializing in different things, not having every [study] try to do exactly the same thing."
• *Comparability* among studies.
• *Data publicly available.* Among researchers and scholars in the social

and economic area, "nobody owns any data. And that is the way it ought to be across the board."

• *Continuity.* "We need to have planning so that we are always getting new data. We are only *beginning* at the beginning of people's lives, and we will need to be able to reap the harvest regularly and not on the basis of occasional one-shot expenditures."

Investments in Research and Intervention at the Community Level

S. Leonard Syme
University of California, Berkeley

We "need to think more creatively about the prevention of disease and promotion of health," Dr. Syme said. In particular, we must make two major innovations: classify diseases not just in terms of their clinical presentation but by their psychosocial precursors and focus not only on the individual but the community. To do so, however, will "require a fundamentally different way of funding research and training programs" from what is currently the norm.

Our identifications of disease risk factors have been based entirely on a clinical model of disease. Taking coronary heart disease as an example, he said, "we have done a good job of identifying several important risk factors for this disease. We all know the list: serum cholesterol, other blood lipids, blood pressure, cigarette smoking, diabetes, physical activity, and so on. [But] the problem is that over half the cases of coronary heart disease are not explained by any of these factors." Though we will undoubtedly discover new risk factors, he said, "I suggest the problem is a more fundamental one. . . . This way of classifying disease is of obvious importance for diagnosing and treating sick people. . . . But is it relevant for *preventing* disease?"

We might take a cue from infectious disease epidemiologists, Dr. Syme said, who "many years ago developed a very different and very successful classification system based on the modes of transmission—waterborne diseases, foodborne diseases, airborne diseases, vectorborne diseases—that different clinical entities had in common. This scheme was not useful in the diagnosis and treatment of sick individuals. But it *was* useful in helping to understand where in the environment disease was coming from, and it was certainly helpful in directing prevention programs."

We do not have an equivalent prevention-oriented classification scheme for the noninfectious diseases we are concerned about today, Dr. Syme maintained, and this issue is of particular importance in the social and behavioral sciences. "Many of the social risk factors we have identified are related not just to one or two clinical diseases but to a long list." We need to study the ways in which these risk factors interact in "compromising the body's defense systems rather than in causing specific diseases. We have been trained to study one clinical disease at a time from one disciplinary perspective, and this may be the reason why our search for risk factors to explain disease occurrence may be less than 100 percent successful."

Unfortunately, he said, "the precise measurement of psychosocial factors is very difficult because the diseases we study are the end result of a very complex series of biological processes. Disease is a very distal consequence of the psychosocial factors under study." But if we could "continue the progress that is now being made in studying such biological concepts as allostatic load or other similar intermediate disease processes, we might be able to improve this situation," Dr. Syme said. "By studying the relationship of psychosocial factors to these more proximal outcomes, two important advances could be made. One advance is that we would have for the first time a disease-related yardstick to help define psychosocial variables more precisely.

"The second advance would be in moving closer to a more appropriate disease classification system. This would help us understand how certain social factors—poverty, social isolation, and particular types of job stress, for example—make people vulnerable to a variety of diseases. And it would help us to think in a way that is more oriented toward disease prevention. It would also provide a useful and efficient way to evaluate the effectiveness of interventions. Instead of having to wait five or 10 years for enough disease to develop in the intervened-upon group, we would be able to observe physiologic changes much sooner."

Our tendency in the health sciences is to focus on individuals rather than the communities in which people live. "As has been demonstrated in many of the presentations at this symposium, we are making important progress in helping people change their behavior to lower their risk of disease," Dr. Syme said. "This is good. But it is important to recognize another dimension of this issue. Even as high-risk people change their behavior and lower their disease risk, new people enter the population to take their places—forever. This is because we rarely identify and take action on those forces in the population that cause the problem in the first place."

To work at the level of the job or the community, we need to develop job- and community-based intervention programs *as well as* individually oriented ones, he maintained. "It is not a question of one approach versus the other; we need to consider both."

Cigarette smoking offers a good example of working at both levels, Dr. Syme said. "We have had phenomenal success, as Margaret Chesney noted, in reducing the prevalence of cigarette smoking—from a mid-40 percent level to around 20 percent today. Part of that success was due to better research on the biology of addiction, and part was due to better clinical treatment methods, both individual and group. But a major part of the success was due to the increased taxes on cigarettes, restrictions on cigarette advertising in magazines and on television, no-smoking laws in public buildings, prohibitions about cigarette sales to minors, changes in the culture about the desirability of smoking, and so on."

Research and intervention programs should be based on an "ecological" model, Dr. Syme said. "This model assumes the differences in level of health and well-being are affected by a dynamic interaction among biologic, behavioral, and environmental forces—an interaction that unfolds over the life course of individuals, families, and communities. This model further assumes that age, gender, race and ethnicity, and socioeconomic differences shape the context in which individuals function and that they therefore directly and indirectly influence health risks and resources.

"An intervention directed to the behavior of adolescents, for example, should take into account not only the adolescents themselves but the environments in which they live, including peer norms, social and neighborhood supports, and ties to community institutions. Similarly, workplace interventions should consider not only the individual attributes of workers but social supports, family and neighborhood influences, environmental and social practices, and so on."

Essential to such interventions and in fact the "common denominator" in our successful efforts, Dr. Syme said, "is that they are multidisciplinary and multilevel in approach." He offered the analogy of designing an airplane, a project that necessarily involves people from hundreds of different disciplines who do not have the option of refusing to interact with one another or to work across disciplinary boundaries. "They have a job to do," he said, and "they need to pool whatever skills and talents they have to accomplish their goal. They *must* work across disciplinary boundaries and at many levels.

"We in the health field have a difficult time behaving in a similar way," Dr. Syme observed. Influenced by the traditions of academia, professionals are organized by discipline, and they tend to stick to their own kind. "There is not as much interdisciplinary interaction as might be expected or hoped for," he said, "and our students of course note this and eventually emulate it in their own lives."

The way we fund research and training programs perpetuates, even encourages, this tradition, Dr. Syme said. "We will not, in my view, begin to deal with this problem until we are able to offer financial incentives to the university to bridge disciplinary perspectives."

But there are already some steps in the right direction, he noted. The counterpart of National Institutes of Health (NIH) in Canada, called the National Institutes of Health Research, not only "contains institutes on heart disease and cancer and arthritis but has also established new institutes that cross disease lines, such as the Institute of Population Health, Institute on Gender, and Institute of Aboriginal Health. . . . And the funding for these institutes is, importantly, determined by the degree to which each institute collaborates with the other institutes."

In a similar spirit, "the Robert Wood Johnson Foundation is currently soliciting proposals from universities to train a generation of population health scholars," Dr. Syme noted. "The emphasis in this program would be on the degree to which universities can develop truly interdisciplinary programs directed toward community health issues."

He acknowledged as well the MacArthur Foundation Network groups and referred to "other beginning initiatives, at both government and foundation levels, that think in terms of community and environmental prevention programs. But all of these efforts are at the very early stages, and funding is still quite limited."

Dr. Syme reminded his audience that "as the population of the United States continues to grow, and to age, the burden of providing appropriate medical care will grow exponentially." Given that our medical care system is already strained, unless we "take more seriously the issue of prevention, and especially *community-based* prevention programs, . . . it is fair to say we ain't seen nuthin' yet."

Reactor Panel for Research Funders

Lynda A. Anderson
Centers for Disease Control and Prevention

"As the Centers for Disease Control and Prevention (CDC) has expanded the scope of its prevention research," Dr. Anderson began, "it has recognized the contributions of the behavioral and social sciences." This important symposium, she thus noted, "will contribute to CDC's continued commitment to prevention research."

Her remarks today, Dr. Anderson said, would focus on two pertinent CDC activities: the Behavioral and Social Science Working Group (BSSWG) and the Prevention Research Centers (PRC) Program.

"Like this symposium," she said, "the BSSWG facilitates communication, collaboration, and partnerships among CDC's social and behavioral scientists." Such agencies "tend to be organized around diseases rather than behavioral issues," she noted, but "since I joined CDC 10 years ago, I have observed a substantial increase in its [more broadly based] behavioral and social research."

BSSWG's membership has grown to more than 200, Dr. Anderson observed, but it's clear, "as indicated by several of [this symposium's] featured speakers, that "a major challenge to behavioral and social scientists is acquiring an understanding of other disciplines' vocabularies while keeping up-to-date in their own fields. This challenge is of particular importance to population-based health research, which is influenced by a wide range of disciplines."

The PRC Program, she said, provides one of several types of extramural prevention research funds available through CDC. It "is designed to connect science and public health practice and to improve health promotion and disease prevention efforts" in four ways by:

- focusing on high-priority public health issues;
- conducting rigorous, community-based prevention research with outcomes applicable to public health programs and policies;
- enhancing community partnerships; and
- bridging gaps between scientific knowledge and public health practices.

The PRC Program, Dr. Anderson noted, has grown since 1986, and presently supports 24* PRCs across the United States at schools of public health, medicine, or osteopathy that have accredited preventive medicine residencies. These PRCs, she said, "serve as a national resource for developing prevention strategies and applying those strategies at the community level." For example, PRC investigators in South Carolina, having identified physical activity as a key issue, are "working collaboratively with a community coalition to include physical activity promotion in its strategic plan." They are also helping the coalition expand and connect a number of walking/biking trials.

"One special feature of the PRC program is community participation" in community-based research, Dr. Anderson said, "although it has taken time for trusting relationships to develop between the PRCs and their community partners" across the nation. "Even regarding methodologies of doing research within communities, we need to understand the process of learning *from* the community as well as doing research *with* the community."

Another priority for the PRC Program is to facilitate the application of research findings, she said. "Because insufficient transnational research has been done in the past, CDC is working with several PRCs to understand what contributes to the uptake of research results and to establish new

---

*Since the time of this presentation, two additional PRCs have been awarded, bringing the total to 26 (*http://www.cdc.gov/prc*).

demonstration projects to examine what works in practice. Some of the concepts derive from CDC's prior work on prevention strategies in HIV/ AIDS."

Finally, Dr. Anderson noted, the PRC Program is actively seeking useful feedback. It is "creating an evaluation process, with help from a large independent consulting firm, [to] clarify how to judge the merit, worth, and significance" of the program. "We will use this information to improve our operations and to provide a basis for accountability. We want to define what we expect of the PRCs over the next five years and then set up evaluation strategies to ensure we are meeting these goals."

J. Michael McGinnis
Robert Wood Johnson Foundation

"My dominant impression of today's session," Dr. McGinnis said, "is that its aggregate implications may be profound for the way we develop our strategies for improving health." There is clearly the need for a "paradigm shift" in our understanding of the determinants of health and in the ways we act on them.

He then discussed four issues in particular that he thought were raised by the symposium's discussions: a new vocabulary, the challenges it implies for the research endeavor, the challenges in the *conduct* of research, and the relevant charges to philanthropy in general and to the Robert Wood Johnson Foundation in particular.

New vocabulary. "What we have heard today are terms like social gradients, psychosocial variables, perceived stress, gene-environment interactions, collective efficacy, system cross-talk, allostasis, aggregate burden, resilience, positive health, and salubrious factors," Dr. McGinnis pointed out. These terms have not heretofore been common to the biomedical sciences, but they *are* "most fundamental to the health of populations."

Challenges for research. "If we think of our health determinants in terms of the primary domains of influence—genetic and biological predisposition, social circumstances, environmental exposures, behavioral choices, and access to medical care," he said, "it is very clear that we have not only an obligation to understand to the fullest the within-domain influences that act in each of those areas but, more importantly, the *cross*-domain influences. That is where the action is."

Conduct of research. Activities that are "born of essentially reductionist concepts," Dr. McGinnis said, are "doomed to reductionist applications. We simply can't be that narrow-minded in the way we structure our priorities and our activities." Instead, "our designs have to begin with concepts that are fundamentally integrative in nature." He then discussed six implications of this new reality for the conduct of research—for "the way we go about our business." They are: how the research enterprise should be organized, the time horizons involved, the methodologies, the capacity to sponsor research, the review processes, and the translation of results.

Organization. We "need to organize at least a part of our research endeavor not around single laboratories but around multiple disciplines, . . . in a fashion that allows new insights with a broader view," Dr. McGinnis said.

Time horizons. Similarly, he noted, we must avoid "the limited perspective of myopic lenses," instead adopting time horizons that "extend as far into the future as we can responsibly, reliably, and validly structure."

Methodologies. We need new analytic models to incorporate the multidisciplinary perspectives of researchers.

Capacity. "We clearly need to have a research community," Dr. McGinnis said, "whose comfort level for dealing in a complex environment is higher than the comfort level of most of our research community to date."

Review process. "We need, in effect, a new set of standards [that] is more generous to alien concepts and approaches."

Translation. "Fundamentally, the public is programmed to focus on single diseases and to [employ] the same kind of reductionist model that orients our research community," Dr. McGinnis said. Thus translating the importance of the broader perspectives of interdisciplinary research "has to be very high on our priority list as we look to the future."

Implications for philanthropy. To complement the major funders—largely in the federal government—of research, the philanthropic community has three basic roles: "gap filling (that is, doing what others don't); leveraging (making it easier for others to do what they want to do); and risk (stepping into arenas that are either politically sensitive or seemingly intractable, or for which the frontiers are ill defined)," Dr. McGinnis said.

He mentioned a few projects in this spirit—and "as testimony to the fact that we are committed to working with you in trying to [cultivate] this new ground"—that the Robert Wood Johnson Foundation currently has under way:

- To complement its risk factor orientation but not to abandon it ("we understand quite clearly the importance of some of the risk factors, whether it is tobacco or alcohol or illegal drugs, or certain others with clear and present impact"), the foundation has "added foci on community health—in particular, on the issues of social isolation and social connectedness—and on population health."

- The foundation is developing a new program of Scholars in Health and Society, "which we hope will deepen the instincts and heighten the comfort level of people for interdisciplinary activity," Dr. McGinnis said. It will parallel Robert Wood Johnson's (RWJ's) established clinical scholars program.

- "Taking a cue from our colleagues at the MacArthur Foundation, and hoping to partner with those colleagues, we will be forming a research network around the issues of social isolation and social connectedness" to focus on the basic mechanisms involved and on the translation of research insights into practical applications.

- "To jumpstart that activity, we will be developing a fairly significant community-oriented research program to try methods, in different ways [and] in different settings, for better engaging those who are most estranged in our society—both to improve their lives and, just as importantly, to learn what kinds of techniques might work."

- "We are committed to expanding our investment in methodologies that can be used for drawing from these interdisciplinary activities."

- "And we will be working again with partners on . . . marshaling the social support for a strong and sustained effort in these areas," he said.

"There are clearly different roles for those of us who come at the funding responsibility from different perspectives," Dr. McGinnis concluded. "But common is the obligation to challenge our assumptions about the way we do business. These six reports [of the NRC and IOM that inspired today's session] will be tremendously helpful in that respect, and I give thanks to each of you who played a part in making that happen."

Judy Vaitukaitis
National Institutes of Health

Dr. Vaitukaitis, who is director of the National Center for Research Resources (NCRR), explained that its job is to work with the 26 other components of National Institutes of Health (NIH) to provide "infrastructure" such as technology, shared resources, and biorepositories. "Our responsibility," she said, "is to catalyze research by defining 'rate-limiting reactions'—steps in the disciplinary research process that limit progress." And although her center serves the entire mission of the National Institutes of Health, Dr. Vaitukaitis's remarks at the symposium concentrated on behavioral research.

Program research support is provided competitively through four NCRR divisions: clinical research, biomedical technology, comparative medicine, and research infrastructure. The Division of Clinical Research is the primary source for behavioral studies and accounts for about two-thirds of NCRR's support in this area: in FY 2001, the division provided approximately $58 million to host behavioral research and that level is estimated to grow to $66 million for the next fiscal year, she said.

The major programs through which NCRR supports behavioral research are the general clinical research centers, approximately 65 biomedical research technology centers, regional primate research centers, and a program for shared instrumentation.

A national network of 80 general clinical research centers (which conduct both inpatient and outpatient research) provides biostatistical support to investigators. The Division of Comparative Medicine supplies animal models of human disease for research. Through the Division of Research Infrastructure, NCRR provides competing grant awards, ranging from $500,000 to $3 million, for the following purposes: building or renovating research laboratories; enhancing the biomedical-research capacity of minority institutions that award Ph.D.s in the health-related disciplines; and supporting eligible institutions in states that receive less than 5 to 7 percent of NIH's grant awards per year.

Examples of clinical research studies "include those on nutrition, exercise, sleep, lifestyle changes, compliance with treatment regimens, and behavioral aspects of unintended pregnancies and transmission of sexually transmitted diseases," Dr. Vaitukaitis said. "We provide the research nurses, the biostatisticians, the specialized laboratories, at no cost to the investigator or to the research subject." (She reminded the audience that NCRR's support is limited to infrastructural resources; "the other parts of NIH— the categoric, or disease-of-the-week institutes—provide the primary research funding to the investigators.")

Clinical research studies "can be carried out longitudinally for long periods of time," Dr. Vaitukaitis observed. "We have many centers that have been in place for more than 30 years, so we match up with the need for longitudinal studies and can probably cut your costs where you use some of these resources."

NCRR also provides access to imaging technologies—"bio-informatics"—and it is in the process of setting up bioinformatics regional centers. "Hearing comments today, it sounds as if you would be good candidates," she said. A consensus derived from the six NRC and IOM reports "would be very helpful to us in moving forward with those bioinformatics resources and being responsive to your needs as well."

Also with respect to imaging research, NCRR is in the process of building a pilot test bed, known as the Biomedical Informatics Network (BIRN), she said, in collaboration with the National Science Foundation, the San Diego Supercomputer Center, and several universities. The BIRN will initially concentrate on neuroscience studies that generate large data objects and host very large databases; this is expected to challenge the network and help drive the development of tools to facilitate sharing of data and its analysis.

"That approach will facilitate the kind of research that some of you have talked about—putting data into a national database so that investigators can access it to do their own research," Dr. Vaitukaitis said. "After getting the bugs out of the system and some sense of what it is going to cost, we will distribute it to the entire country so that any behavioral, biomedical, or basic-science investigators supported by other federal agencies or the private sector would be able to have access."

With regard to animal models, "mouse models for a variety of diseases and genetic modifications are available" from NCRR, she said. "We support Jackson Labs and have recently started a national *network* of Jackson Labs, if you will, for this purpose."

She also noted that NCRR is in the process of working with NIH's Genome Institute to develop the rhesus monkey as a model for polygenic disorders. "The technology to be developed over the next couple of years is intended to examine risk factors, such as drugs or environmental exposures, that modulate gene function. The nonhuman primate can also be used for studying neurodegenerative and other diseases."

The resources described above are just a sample of NCRR's repertoire, selected to address some of the research needs relevant to this symposium, Dr. Vaitukaitis said. They are merely the tip of the iceberg.

"The president's budget request for NCRR is just under a billion dollars. NCRR's role is to be a catalyst for discovery—to find out what researchers' needs are and then to set priorities with the collective community to address the most pressing needs first."

Wrap-up

Kenneth I. Shine
Institute of Medicine

"A little over four years ago, a group of about a dozen of us gathered together on a Sunday to discuss with Harold Varmus what might happen in the course of a doubling of the National Institutes of Health (NIH) budget, and I raised a question about NIH's investment in the social and behavioral sciences," Dr. Shine began. "Harold's response was: 'I understand where the frontiers are in research in genomics. I *don't know* where the frontiers are in research in the social and behavioral sciences.' "

His comment was not a hostile one, Dr. Shine recalled; he was simply asking for guidance. In response, several projects have since been undertaken to help enlighten such influential decisionmakers: the report titled *Promoting Health: Intervention Strategies from Social and Behavioral Research* supported by the Woodruff Foundation; the six National Research Council and Institute of Medicine reports, supported by NIH, Center for Disease Control (CDC), and the Robert Wood Johnson Foundation, that are the basis of this symposium; and continuing efforts by the National Research Council (NRC) and the Institute of Medicine (IOM) "in both the research and practice of what we need to do with regard to the social and behavioral sciences."

IOM's projects in these areas that are currently underway include a congressionally mandated study on racial disparities; a study on the vision of public health for the 21st century; a congressionally mandated study on the structure of the NIH with regard to existing institutes, their relationships to one another, and additional kinds of programs; and a project on health communication.

Today's presentations are themselves important contributions to delineating the frontiers of research in the social and behavioral sciences, Dr. Shine said, and he proceeded to share some of his reactions to them.

First, he agreed that multidisciplinary efforts—essential if the social and behavioral sciences are truly to have an impact on health—imply the need to learn a new vocabulary. Terms like social network, social ecology, norms, ecometrics, and allostatic loads can be confusing for those who are not experts in their respective fields of origin. Thus "one of the greatest challenges," Dr. Shine said, will be in "making the language more explicit and more precise and to increase the amount of common understanding."

He observed that even in the course of producing the six NRC and IOM reports, "I was struck, in the deliberations of the committees, by the number of times in which there were either misunderstandings of language or unwillingness to accept particular *uses* of language—particularly among individuals coming to the problem from different disciplines." That being the case, he added, imagine "the problem of how the public, or funders, or policymakers are going to understand what you're talking about."

The need to simplify, clarify, and generally improve the quality of communication is particularly important at the interface between social/behavioral sciences and biology, Dr. Shine said. "There are major obstacles here, as we talk with each other, about what we mean in terms of hypotheses, methods, and research design."

And it's essential that a sense of audience also pervade communication with potential patrons, he noted. For example, though the need for "multilayered comprehensive approaches"—a term that has appropriately come up at this symposium—is indisputable, "I hope that nobody tries to convince a congressional committee that there ought to be more funding for [studies] based on multilayered comprehensive approaches." The challenge is to show that need, clearly and concretely.

Other challenges mentioned at this symposium that we need to keep in mind include maintenance and scaling-up, Dr. Shine said. For example, "I'd like to know, in a weight reduction intervention in the community, how long that lasted" after the activities—often requiring an enormous investment of time, effort, and energy—were terminated.

Similarly, he continued, we have a major problem with scaling-up—in generalizing—activities. "We do a very good job with isolated projects, usually around an enthusiastic or charismatic leader," he said. But it's striking how often that leader's presence *determines* the outcome, which we are then unable to duplicate. "We need to ask ourselves, in every case where we fund an activity: What is the essence of it that will allow it to be generalized? And what would be its requirements? And what would be required to maintain it?"

There was some discussion today about the "magnitude of change," Dr. Shine said, and "that is a very, very, very important concept." If, for example, we wring our hands that certain interventions at reducing substance abuse—say, involving cocaine or heroin—have "only" increased the number of cures from 12 to 20 percent, that completely misses the social and individual value of having almost twice as many people who are now drug-free. Similarly, improving the vaccination rate for the nation by "only" 2 or 3 percent may seem marginal, "but in terms of the number of human lives that are affected, that is spectacular. And if it's your kid, it's your whole world. We need to address that issue and to communicate it much more effectively," he said.

Although Dr. Shine agreed that *multiple* interventions are often needed, there still has to be some sense of priority setting. "We don't have the resources to do everything," he said, so we need to distinguish the questions that can be answered from those that cannot. For example, at-risk populations often merit high priority not only for reasons of equity, morality, or compassion, but also because they provide a mechanism for asking clearer questions and getting clearer answers.

Another illustration of priority setting: "You may be aware that 20 conditions account for 80 percent of health care expenditures in the United States," Dr. Shine said; IOM has recommended 15 of those to be targets. Each of the targets should entail treatment and prevention approaches geared to individuals, along with public health, population-based strategies. And each orientation complements the other. "We believe that focusing on integrated care, care systems, and multidisciplinary care has the potential to create resonance with some of the things we are talking about in public health," he said.

Meanwhile, Dr. Shine noted, "our discussions with medical school deans, accrediting organizations, and others [who examine physicians] is that there ought to be increased training in population issues and prevention" because "clearly we are too far over on the individual side." Still, he cautioned, "this is not about populations versus individuals. It is about populations *and* individuals. Figuring out how to balance that and where the resources are to go obviously requires a resetting, if you will, of the thermostat."

Another needed balance is between reductionism and integration. "The 20th century was, and maybe the first decade of the 21st century will be, a continuation of the biomedical reductionist approach," he said. "But biomedicine is already beginning to turn the corner. Once you start talking about gene products, protein structure, the structure of cells, the structure of organs, the mind in terms of neuroscience, you will see serious integration beginning to take place."

There are some synergisms here that we should take advantage of, Dr. Shine said. "Those in public health need to piggyback to some extent on what happens in biomedicine and the health care delivery system, and those in biomedicine and the health care delivery system need to work with colleagues in public health, and not make this an either-or kind of a proposition."

But with regard to another trade-off mentioned at this symposium—of advocacy versus science—Dr. Shine urged researchers to stick with science. "An enormous problem in the entire field of the social and behavioral sciences arises from the notion that we mix everything into it—poverty, income redistribution, all kinds of stuff that has political connotations," he said. "But the best way we can address these kinds of problems is by doing the very best science—objective, well-placed, evidence-based science." Providing such solid analysis will in the long run be far more persuasive to the media, the public, and its leaders, he insisted, than when researchers complicate matters by inserting themselves into the political process.

Mixing beliefs with facts can cause complications even closer to home. The six NRC and IOM studies we have talked about today were not easy to do, Dr. Shine noted. In fact, he considered them to be among the hardest studies he has been involved with during his nine and a half years at IOM. "As I look back at why they were hard, it wasn't because the data were not sufficient," he said, "but because many of the people on our committees—and God bless all of them, 104 plus the chairs; they did a splendid job—came with belief systems that may or may not have been based on data."

Referring to his point about language at the beginning of these remarks, Dr. Shine concluded, "It is very important that we enhance our understanding of each other, and that in our deliberations we work very hard to look at the data."

Appendix A: Symposium Agenda

Through the Kaleidoscope:
Viewing the Contributions of the Behavioral and
Social Sciences to Health
The Barbara and Jerome Grossman Symposium: 2001

National Academy of Sciences
2101 Constitution Avenue, N.W.
Washington, D.C. 20418

May 23, 2001

8:00 am   **Continental Breakfast**

9:00 am   **Welcome**
Jerome H. Grossman, M.D., Senior Fellow for the Health Care
Delivery Project, Kennedy School of Government, Harvard
University

9:10 am   **Introduction to the Subject**
Lisa F. Berkman, Ph.D., Chair, Department of Health and
Social Behavior, Florence Sprague Norman and Laura Smart
Norman Professor of Health and Social Behavior, Harvard
School of Public Health, Harvard University

Scholarship in the behavioral and social sciences has made
significant strides over the last decade and is poised to
assume a central role in understanding and influencing the
determinants of health. Realizing that opportunity
requires bold new thinking in research design, training,
infrastructure investments, and grant making.

9:35 am   **What We Know: The Tantalizing Potential**
           Etiology, Part I
           John Cacioppo, Ph.D., Tiffany and Margaret Blake
           Distinguished Service Professor; Director, Social Psychology
           Program; and Co-Director, Institute for Mind and Biology,
           The University of Chicago

           Etiology, Part II
           Robert J. Sampson, Ph.D., Lucy Flower Professor in Sociology,
           Department of Social Sciences, The University of Chicago

10:15 am   **Q&A**

10:25 am   **Early Childhood Interventions: Theories of Change,**
           Empirical Findings, and Research Priorities
           Interventions, Part I
           Jack P. Shonkoff, M.D., Dean, Heller Graduate School;
           Samuel F. and Rose B. Gingold Professor of Human
           Development and Social Policy, Brandeis University

           Interventions, Part II
           Margaret Chesney, Ph.D., Professor of Medicine, Professor of
           Epidemiology and Biostatistics, School of Medicine,
           University of California, San Francisco

11:05 am   **Q&A**

11:15 am   **Why Exploiting This Knowledge Will Be Essential to**
           Achieving Health Improvements in the 21st Century
           Raynard S. Kington, M.D., Ph.D., Associate Director
           of Behavioral and Social Sciences Research, National
           Institutes of Health

11:45 am   **Q&A**

12:00 pm   **Lunch**

1:00 pm   **Refocus**
             Lisa F. Berkman, Ph.D., Harvard School of Public Health

             Priority investments necessary to support rapid advances in
             the behavioral and social sciences.

1:15 pm   **Research to Understand the Mechanisms Through Which
             Social and Behavioral Factors Influence Health**
             Bruce S. McEwen, Ph.D., Alfred E. Mirsky Professor, Harold
             and Margaret Milliken Hatch Laboratory of
             Neuroendocrinology, The Rockefeller University

1:45 pm   **Q&A**

2:00 pm   **Investments in Longitudinal Surveys, Databases,
             Advanced Statistical Research, and Computation
             Technology**
             Robert M. Hauser, M.D., Vilas Research Professor of
             Sociology, Center for Demography of Health and Aging,
             University of Wisconsin

2:30 pm   **Q&A**

2:45 pm   **Investments in Research and Interventions at the
             Community Level**
             S. Leonard Syme, Ph.D., Professor Emeritus, Division of
             Public Health Biology and Epidemiology, University of
             California, Berkeley

3:15 pm   **Q&A**

3:30 pm   **Reactor Panel for Research Funders**
             Lynda A. Anderson, Ph.D., Senior Health Scientist, Prevention
             Research Centers Program, National Center for Chronic
             Disease Prevention and Health Promotion, Centers for
             Disease Control and Prevention

J. Michael McGinnis, M.D., Senior Vice President and Director, Health Group, Robert Wood Johnson Foundation

Judy Vaitukaitis, M.D., Director, National Center for Research Resources, National Institutes of Health

4:10 pm   **Wrap-up**

Kenneth I. Shine, M.D., President, Institute of Medicine